Copyright ©2021 THEO WILLIAMS MD
All rights reserved. No part of this publication may be reproduced, distributed, or transmitted in any form or by any means, including photocopying, recording, or other electronic or mechanical methods, without the prior written permission of the publisher, except in the case of brief quotations embodied in critical reviews and certain other noncommercial uses permitted by copyright law.

Contents

Introduction 3

Categories of Dog food 5

Dry Food..5

Dry food Manufacturing process 6

Wet food 8

Wet food Manufacturing Process 9

Semi-Moist food..10

Alternatives 11

What are the Options?..12

Ingredients to Avoid 15

Calcium..15

Dog Food Add-Ins 15

Making the Switch 16

One Size Fits All? 17

Allergy Alternatives 18

Quality, Digestibility And Energy Density 19

Labeling...20

Types of Diets..22

Senior Dog Diet 23

Low-protein Dog diet 26

Disadvantages of Low Diet 27

Advantages of Low Diet 28

Hypoallergenic diet 29

Grain-free and low-carbohydrate diet 31

Vegetarian and Vegan dog diet 33

Nutrients and Supplements 35

Foods Dangerous to Dogs 35

Contaminants 36

Common Mistakes When Cooking For Your Dog 38

An Alternative To Home Cooking 41

Conclusion 42

Introduction

As dog owners, we are often advised not to share our meals with our dogs. So what do we cook for our them? Many human ingredients are actually fine. The difference is that food we prepare for ourselves often contains elements that aren't friendly to our dogs, or are too rich or fatty for their systems. Using healthy ingredients to prepare food meant for their systems is just fine. Variety is key! Cooking at home for your dog offers what commercially bought food cannot, and that is an assortment of flavors and textures. More importantly, it offers a variety of vitamins and nutrients that you might not get in a bag of dog food. You can mix and match ingredients, offering a host of flavors for your canine while meeting his nutritional needs. Not to mention he'll be one happy dog!

Dog food is food specifically formulated and intended for consumption by dogs and other related canines. Dogs are considered to be omnivores with a carnivorous bias. They have the sharp, pointed teeth and shorter gastrointestinal tracts of carnivores, better suited for the consumption of meat than of vegetable substances, yet also have 10 genes that are responsible for starch and glucose digestion, as well as the ability to produce amylase, an enzyme that functions to break down carbohydrates into simple sugars - something that carnivores lack. Dogs evolved the ability living alongside humans in agricultural societies, as they managed on scrap leftovers from humans.

Categories of Dog food

Dry Food

Dry dog food usually consists of bagged kibble that contains 3-11% water. It makes up the vast majority of pet foods. Dry food is both convenient and typically inexpensive, with over $8 billion worth being sold in 2010 – a 50% increase over just seven years earlier.

Dry dog food considerations

Advantages:

- Ease of storage and feeding
- Energy-dense
- Cost effective More likely to contain preservatives

Disadvantages:

- Lower palatability when compared to wet food

- Often contains more grains, which may be undesirable for dogs with allergies
- More likely to contain preservatives

Dry food Manufacturing process

Dry food processing is popular in the pet food industry, as it is an efficient way to supply continuous production of feed in many varieties. It is energy efficient, allows for large amounts of feed to be used, and is cost effective.

To make dog kibble, a process known as extrusion is done. A simple extruder consists of a barrel, helical screws, and a die (tool to cut and shape food). Feed ingredients are solid at room temperature; therefore, the extrusion process of these ingredients requires a temperature above 150 degrees Celsius, achieved by the use of steam, hot water, or other heat sources in order to soften or melt the mixture and allow for fluidity through the barrel.

During the extrusion process, the high amounts of pressure applied to the mixture forces it to enter through the die before exiting the extruder completely, where it is cut to its desired size by a rotating fly knife.

Unfortunately, the extrusion process actually denatures some of nutritional elements of the food. Taurine deficiency has been found in dogs and cats fed extruded commercial diets. Not usually considered an essential nutrient for dogs, taurine is plentiful in most whole meats, whether raw or cooked, but is reduced in extruded diets. Taurine deficiency could also be due to the use of rendered, highly processed meat sources that are low in taurine. Regardless of the cause, taurine is now artificially supplemented back into the diet after processing in the production of most commercial pet food.

Wet food

Wet or canned dog food usually is packaged in a solid or soft-sided container. Wet food contains roughly 60-78% water, which is significantly higher in moisture than dry or semi-moist food. Canned food is commercially sterile (cooked during canning); other wet foods may not be sterile. Sterilizing is done through the process of retorting, which involves steam sterilization at 121 degrees Celsius.

A given wet food will often be higher in protein or fat compared to a similar kibble on a dry matter basis (a measure which ignores moisture); given the canned food's high moisture content, however, a larger amount of canned food must be fed in order to meet the dog's required energy needs. Grain gluten and other protein gels may be used in wet dog food to create artificial meaty chunks, which look like real meat. This food is usually used for old dogs or puppies.

Wet dog food considerations

Advantages:

- Increased palatability
- Often higher in protein and fat
- Easier to eat

Disadvantages:

- Spoilage
- Expensive
- Linked to weight gain

Wet food Manufacturing Process

After ingredients are combined, they are placed in a tank at the end of a canning machine. From there, the mixture is forced through an opening and onto a metal sheet, forming a thickness of 8 to 12mm.[29] Next, the mixture is heated to thoroughly cook the ingredients. Heating can be done through the means of ovens, microwaves or steam heating.

The sheet containing a layer of feed is passed through the heat source that displays heat to the top and bottom of the tray, allowing the internal temperature to reach 77 degrees Celsius at a minimum. Once cooked, this mixture can be directly placed into cans to form a loaf or it can be cut into "meaty" pieces for chunks and gravy formulas.

Semi-Moist food

Semi-moist dog food is packaged in vacuum-sealed pouches or packets. It contains about 20-45% water by weight, making it more expensive per energy calorie than dry food.

Semi-moist dog food considerations

Advantages:

- Energy-dense
- High Palability
- Convenient

Advantages:

- Contains artificial color, chemical preservatives, and chemical flavor enhancer
- Contains higher levels of sodium and sugar
- Expensive

Most semi-moist food does not require refrigeration. They are lightly cooked and then quickly sealed in a vacuum package. This type of dog food is extremely vulnerable to spoiling if not kept at a cool temperature and has a shelf life of 2–4 months, unopened.

Alternatives

Some alternatives to traditional commercial pet foods are available. Many companies have been successful in targeting niche markets, each with unique characteristics. Some popular alternative dog food types are:

Dehydrated or freeze-dried meals come in raw and cooked forms. Products are usually air-dried or frozen, then dehydrated (freeze-dried) to reduce moisture to the level where bacterial growths are inhibited. The appearance is very similar to dry kibbles. The typical feeding methods include adding warm water before serving. There is some concern of nutrients, such as vitamins, being lost during the dehydration process.

Specialty "small batch" type feeds sold through specialty or online stores generally consist of some form of cooked meat, ground bone, pureed vegetables, taurine supplements, and other multivitamin supplements. Some pet owners use human vitamin supplements, and others use vitamin supplements specifically engineered for dogs.

What are the Options?

You don't have to prepare all of your dog's food. You can also provide a mixture of healthy commercial dog food with add-ins of your own healthy ingredients. Here are some of the ingredients to use and what to stay away:

- Protein

You might assume that cooking for your dog means primarily protein. Dogs are like us, though, in that they need a healthy balance of protein, carbohydrates and veggies. A balance between these elements is essential, but it can vary between dogs.

A good recommendation is 40% protein, 50% vegetables and 10% starch. Some dogs cannot handle high amounts of protein, though, so it is important to visit your vet to determine the best ratio to suit their dietary needs. Beef, Turkey, Chicken, Lamb, Pork, Shrimp (fully cooked with shell removed), Tuna, Eggs (in moderation)

Avoid cuts of meat that are too fatty or rich, or covered in garlic or seasonings. Remove excess fat and skin, and watch for poultry bones which can splinter. Use meats like ham in moderation which are usually high in sodium and fat.

- Vegetables

Carrots, Green beans, Spinach, Peas Celery, Cucumbers, Pumpkin, Sweet Potato, Corn

- Carbohydrates

Rice, Potatoes, Pasta, Oatmeal, Quinoa (Within limits since these have limited nutritional value.)

- Other Foods

Coconut, coconut milk and coconut oil. Honey. Fruits such as strawberries, raspberries, apples, pineapple, and melon. Peanuts and peanut butter are okay in moderation. Avoid salted peanuts. Unsalted, unbuttered, air-popped popcorn is okay in moderation. Watch for unpopped kernels.

Ingredients to Avoid

Alcohol, Almonds, Avocados, Chocolate, Coffee, Cinnamon, Garlic, Grapes, Onions, Macadamia nuts, Raisins, Raw yeast dough, Xylitol and artificial sweeteners, and Mushrooms are some of the ingredients to avoid.

Calcium

Don't forget the calcium! Ingredients such as cottage cheese or plain yogurt are great paired with fruits which offer vitamins and antioxidants. You can offer this as a treat throughout the day or you can include it in their meal. Watch for signs such as vomiting or diarrhea as some pups are lactose intolerant. Avoid or use caution with amounts for higher-fat options like ice cream and cheese.

Dog Food Add-Ins

If you prefer to feed your dog a mixture of kibble with add-ins, some good options would be:

- a whole egg (you can give it raw or you can cook it)
- a can of cooked salmon
- mixed vegetables raw or steamed
- a small portion of cottage cheese or yogurt
- leafy greens such as kale or spinach (helps to digest the kibble)

Making the Switch

A good thing to remember is that most dogs cannot switch overnight from store-bought dog food to home cooked food. It's best to transition slowly over a period of 6 days to a week.

- Day 1 – Mix 20% of the new food with 80% of the old.
- Day 2 – Mix 40% of the new food with 60% of the old.
- Day 3 – Mix 50% of the new food with 50% of the old
- Day 4 – Mix 60% of the new food with 40% of the old.

- Day 5 – Mix 80% of the new food with 20% of the old.
- Day 6 – Feed 100% of the new food.

Keep an eye out for any health concerns such as diarrhea, vomiting or lack of eating. If you see digestive issues, either back off the transition, see if you can identify what food your dog has an issue with, or contact your veterinarian.

One Size Fits All?

A Chihuahua and a Great Dane certainly do not eat the same amount. Volume and calories still matter when it comes to home-cooked dog food so it's important to know what you're feeding. The best way to start is to look up recipes online that already have ingredient information until you feel more comfortable about portions. It's a good practice to show your veterinarian the recipes you've prepared (or plan to prepare) to be sure they meet your pup's needs. Also ask your veterinarian to recommend a multivitamin supplement and a mineral supplement to make sure your dog is getting the appropriate amt of calcium, phosphorus, etc.

Also, weigh your pup regularly to be sure they maintain a healthy weight. This can be done at home or at the vet's office. If you're unsure of what a healthy weight range would be for your dog, check with your veterinarian. And preparing tasty dog food at home is also a healthy way to help your dog shed extra pounds. We don't recommend obsessing over calories–just learning the basics and ensuring that your pup's health stays on track.

We also don't recommend a home-cooked diet for dogs under a year of age because if not given the correct amounts of calcium and phosphorus, a young dog could develop significant bone abnormalities.

Allergy Alternatives

Switching to home-cooked can take time a little time to find the right balance but it isn't overly complicated. But, many dogs have individual food preferences, as well as food allergies. At first, you will need to monitor whether your pup is allergic to certain ingredients.

At Union Lake Veterinary Hospital, we encourage and support a healthy diet for your pets. If you have nutrition or diet questions on what is best for them, give us a call or set up an appointment any time!

Quality, Digestibility And Energy Density

There are a few key components to consider when evaluating dietary needs. These factors include the quality and digestibility of the protein provided in the diet, as well as the composition of the amino acids included, and finally the energy density provided in the diet.

Diets containing proteins that are high in quality, composition, and digestibility require less of that protein to be present. The same can be said in regards to the energy density. In contrast, high-protein diets will provide excess protein content after meeting maintenance demands; this can therefore lead to the protein being utilized in fat and energy storage.

This ultimately increases the risk for developing obesity and other health related issues. However, higher protein in the diet helps reduce lean body mass loss, but will not lead to an increase in size of muscle unless paired with resistance exercises or anabolic steroids under maintenance conditions.

Labeling

Further information: Pet food § Labeling and regulation

In the United States, dog foods labelled as "complete and balanced" must meet standards established by the Association of American Feed Control Officials (AAFCO), either by meeting a nutrient profile or by passing a feeding trial. The Dog Food Nutrient Profiles were last updated in 2016 by the AAFCO's Canine Nutrition Expert Subcommittee.

Critics argue that due to the limitations of the trial and the gaps in knowledge within animal nutrition science, the term "complete and balanced" is inaccurate and even deceptive. An AAFCO panel expert has stated that "although the AAFCO profiles are better than nothing, they provide false securities."

Certain manufacturers label their products with terms such as "premium", "ultra premium", "natural", and "holistic". Such terms currently have no legal definitions and are not regulated. There are also varieties of dog food labeled as "human-grade food." Although no official definition of this term exists, the assumption is that other brands use foods that would not pass US Food and Drug Administration inspection according to the Pure Food and Drug Act or the Meat Inspection Act.

The ingredients on the label must be listed in descending order by weight before cooking. This means before all of the moisture is removed from the meat, fruits, vegetables and other ingredients used.

Types of Diets

Raw feeding is the practice of feeding domestic dogs, cats and other animals a diet consisting primarily of uncooked meat, edible bones, and organs. The ingredients used to formulate raw diets can vary. Some pet owners choose to make homemade raw diets to feed their animals but commercial raw food diets are also available.

Frozen, or fresh-prepared, meals come in raw or cooked form, some of which is made with ingredients that are inspected, approved, and certified by the USDA for human consumption, but formulated for pets. Part of this growing trend is the commercialization of home-made dog food for pet owners who want the same quality, but do not have the time or expertise to make it themselves. The advantage is forgoing the processing stage that traditional dog food undergoes. This causes less destruction of its nutritional integrity.

The practice of feeding raw diets has raised some concerns due to the risk of foodborne illnesses, zoonosis and nutritional imbalances. People who feed their dogs raw food do so for a multitude of reasons, including but not limited to: culture, beliefs surrounding health, nutrition and what is perceived to be more natural for their pets. Feeding raw food can be perceived as allowing the pet to stay in touch with their wild, carnivorous ancestry.[51] The raw food movement has occurred in parallel to the change in human food trends for more natural and organic products.

Senior Dog Diet

Senior dogs require specialized diets that are catered towards the aging animal. There are various physiological changes which a dog goes through as it ages. Commercially available senior dog diets address these changes through various ingredients and nutrients.

When looking for a senior dog food, one of the first things that should be taken into consideration is the energy content of the diet. The maintenance energy requirements decrease as a dog ages due to the loss in lean body mass that occurs. Therefore, senior dogs will require a diet with a lowered energy content compared to non senior diets. Although senior dogs require lower energy content diets, they will also require diets that are higher in protein and protein digestibility. This is due to the fact that dogs have a reduced ability to synthesize proteins as they age.

Joint and bone health is an important factor to be considered when purchasing a senior dog food. The addition of glucosamine and chondroitin sulfate has been shown to improve cartilage formation, the composition of synovial fluid, as well as improve signs of osteoarthritis. The calcium to phosphorus ratio of senior dog foods is also important. Calcium and phosphorus are considered essential nutrients, according to AAFCO.

Gastrointestinal health is another important factor to consider in the aging dog. Sources of fiber such as beet pulp and flaxseed should be included within senior dog foods to help improve stool quality and prevent constipation.

A current technology that is being used to improve gastrointestinal health of aging dogs is the addition of fructooligosacchardies and mannanoligosaccharides. These oligosaccharides are used in combination to improve the beneficial gut bacteria while eliminating the harmful gut bacteria.

The aging dog goes through changes in brain and cognitive health. There are two highly important ingredients that can be included in senior dog foods to help prevent cognitive decline and improve brain health. These ingredients are vitamin E and L-carnitne. Vitamin E acts as an antioxidant, which can prevent oxidative damage that occurs during aging. L-carnitine is used to improve mitochondrial function, which can also help to prevent and lower rates of oxidative damage.

Skin and coat health is important in all dogs, but especially becomes important as dogs age. An important nutrient to look for in senior dog foods to support coat health is linoleic acid, which can be found in corn and soybean oil. Another important nutrient is vitamin A, which helps with keratinization of hair. Good sources of vitamin A for skin and coat health include egg yolk and liver.

Immune system health has been shown to decline in aging dogs. The ratio of omega-6 to omega-3 fatty acids plays an important role in providing optimal health. Vitamin E can be used as an antioxidant in senior dog foods. Pre- and probiotics can also be added to senior dog foods to help improve the beneficial bacteria in the gut, providing support for the immune system.

Low-protein Dog diet

According to The Association of American Feed Control Officials (AAFCO) nutrient guideline for cats and dogs, the minimum protein requirement for dogs during adult maintenance is 18% on a dry matter (DM) basis. Other parts of the world would have a guideline similar to AAFCO.

The European Pet Food Federation (FEDIAF) also stated a minimum of 18%. AAFCO only provided a minimum, but majority of the diets found on the market contain a protein level exceeding the minimum. Some diets have a protein level lower than others (such as 18-20%). These low-protein diets would not be seen with growth and reproductive life stages because of their higher demand for protein, as such, these diets are for dogs meeting maintenance levels. They can be purchased, such as vegetarian, vegan, weight control, and senior diets. Furthermore, this protein requirement varies from species to species.

Disadvantages of Low Diet

There is an increasing risk of the practice of coprophagy when providing low-protein diets to dogs; a negative correlation exists between the amount of protein fed and the occurrence of coprophagy. Maintenance needs should still be met by low-protein diets, and the muscle turnover (i.e. synthesis and breakdown) will also remain at an optimal rate, as long as the amino acid intake remains balanced and there are no limiting amino acids.However, there is a greater opportunity for amino acids to be balanced in diets containing higher protein content.

Advantages of Low Diet

The dog's simple gastrointestinal tract contains a vast array of microbial populations; some members of this very diversified community include fusobacteria, proteobacteria, and actinobacteria.

The gut microbiota of the dog will be comparable to that of the owners due to similar environmental impacts. Not only are the microbes influenced by the dog's environment, but they are also affected by the macronutrient content of the dog's diet. The populations present and health status of the microbiota found within the gut can alter the physiological and metabolic functions of the dog, which then subsequently affects susceptibility to disease development.

Fermentation and digestion in the hindgut of a dog can potentially be improved depending on the source and the concentration of protein provide in a diet. Greater digestibility due to higher quality ingredients, in addition to lower protein concentrations within a diet, will help promote beneficial outcomes in assisting the health of a dog's gastrointestinal tract. Higher protein entering the gut will lead to more putrefaction that give rise to various toxins including carcinogens and increase the chances of many bowel diseases, such as colorectal cancer.

The age of dogs and cats is inversely proportional to protein consumption. As they age, the protein requirement decreases due to lower level of pepsin in their stomachs. There has also been discussion about higher protein content in diets being inversely related with lifespan (i.e. negative relationship), where lower protein content diets were related to longer lifespans.

Hypoallergenic diet

Dogs are prone to have adverse allergic reactions to food similar to human beings. The most common symptoms of food allergies in dogs include rashes, swelling, itchy or tender skin, and gastrointestinal upsets such as uncontrollable bowel movements and soft stools. Certain ingredients in dog food can elicit these allergic reactions. Specifically, the reactions are understood to be initiated by the protein ingredients in dog food, with sources such as beef, chicken, soy, and turkey being common causes of these allergic reactions. A number of "novel protein" dog foods are available that claim to alleviate such allergies in dogs.

Hypoallergenic diets for dogs with food allergies consist of either limited ingredients, novel proteins or hydrolyzed proteins. Limited ingredients make it possible to identify the suspected allergens causing these allergic reactions, as well as making it easy to avoid multiple ingredients if a canine is allergic to more than one.

In novel protein recipes, manufacturers use ingredients which are less likely to cause allergic reactions in dogs such as lamb, fish, and rice.Hydrolyzed proteins do not come from a novel source; they could originate from chicken or soy for example. Hydrolyzed proteins become novel when they are broken apart into unrecognizable versions of themselves, making them novel to allergic gastrointestinal tracts.

Grain-free and low-carbohydrate diet

Some dog food products differentiate themselves as grain- or carbohydrate-free to offer the consumer an alternative, claiming carbohydrates in pet foods to be fillers with little or no nutritional value. However, a study published in Nature suggests that domestic dogs' ability to easily metabolize carbohydrates may be a key difference between wolves and dogs.

Despite consumer and manufacturer claims that dogs perform better on grain-free diets, many veterinarians doubt their benefits, pointing to a historical lack of research documenting any benefits. In 2019, a study comparing dry dog food that was manufactured in the United States found that 75% of food containing feed grade grains also contained measurable levels of various mycotoxins (discussed below), while none of the grain-free dry diets tested had any detectable levels of mycotoxins.

Feed grade (lower quality grade) grains that are allowed to spoil and become moldy are the suspected source of the mycotoxins. This is the first published study to show a potential health benefit to feeding grain-free commercial dry pet foods.

In 2019, the U.S. Food and Drug Administration identified 16 dog food brands linked to canine heart disease. The FDA has investigated more than 500 cases of dilated cardiomyopathy in dogs eating food marketed as grain-free. The 16 brands are: Acana, Zignature, Taste of the Wild, 4Health, Earthborn Holistic, Blue Buffalo, Nature's Domain, Fromm, Merrick, California Natural, Natural Balance, Orijen, Nature's Variety, NutriSource, Nutro, and Rachael Ray Nutrish. These brands are labeled as "grain-free" and list peas, lentils, or potatoes as the main ingredient. The top three brands associated with reports of cardiomyopathy are Acana with 67 reports, Zignature with 64, and Taste of the Wild with 53 reports.

Vegetarian and Vegan dog diet

Like the human practice of veganism, vegan dog foods are those formulated with the exclusion of ingredients that contain or were processed with any part of an animal, or any animal byproduct. Vegan dog food may incorporate the use of fruits like bananas, vegetables, cereals, legumes, nuts, vegetable oils, or soya, as well as any other non-animal based foods. The omnivorous domestic canine has evolved to metabolize carbohydrates and thrive on a diet lower in protein, and therefore, a vegan diet may be substantial if properly formulated and balanced.

Popularity of this diet has grown with a corresponding increase in people practicing vegetarianism and veganism, and there are now various commercial vegetarian and vegan diets available on the market. Vegetarian dog foods are produced to either assuage a pet owner's ethical concerns or for animals with extreme allergies.

Due to the exclusion of animal products and by-products, which are primary ingredients of conventional dog food, many nutrients that would otherwise be provided by animal products need to be provided by replacement, plant-based ingredients. While both animal and plant products offer a wide range of macro and micronutrients, strategic formulation of plant ingredients should be considered to meet nutritional requirements, as different nutrients are more abundant in different plant sources. Despite the large differences in ingredient sourcing, studies have demonstrated that a plant-based diet can be just as edible and palatable as animal-based diets for dogs.

Some nutrients that require special consideration include protein, calcium, vitamin D, vitamin B12, taurine, L-carnitine, and omega-3 fatty acids, particularly DHA and EPA. Although their sources are more limited without animal products, it is possible to formulate a diet adequate in these nutrients through plant and synthetic sources.

Potential risks in feeding a plant-based diet include alkaline urine and nutrient inadequacy, especially in homemade diets. Adherence to recommendations by reliable sources is strongly advised.

Nutrients and Supplements

The requirements and functions of nutrients in dogs are largely similar to those in cats, with many requirements relaxed:

The requirement of arginine in the urea cycle is reduced, as dogs have a functional pyrroline-5-carboxylate synthase.

- Dogs have a functional delta 6 desaturase, hence no specific need for arachidonic acid.
- Dogs have a function sulfinoalanine decarboxylase, hence no need for taurine.
- Unlike cats, dogs and humans can use Vitamin D2 as efficiently as they use Vitamin D3.

Foods Dangerous to Dogs

A number of common human foods and household ingestibles are toxic to dogs, including chocolate solids (theobromine poisoning), onion and garlic (thiosulfate, sulfoxide or disulfide poisoning), grapes and raisins (cause kidney failure in dogs), milk (some dogs are lactose intolerant and suffer diarrhea; goats' milk can be beneficial), nutmeg (neurotoxic to dogs), mushrooms, fatty foods, rhubarb, xylitol,[97] macadamia nuts, as well as various plants and other potentially ingested materials. A full list of poison/toxic substances can be found on the ASPCA's website.

Contaminants
- Mycotoxins

In April 2014, aflatoxin B1, a known carcinogenic toxin, melamine, and cyanuric acid were all found in various brands of USA pet food imported into Hong Kong. Since 1993, the FDA has confirmed concerns of toxins in feed grade (animal grade) ingredients, yet to date no comprehensive federal regulation exists on mycotoxin testing in feed grade (animal grade) ingredients used to make pet food.

In 1997, the Journal of Food Additives and Contaminants established that low levels of various mycotoxins could cause health concerns in pets, and was found in feed grade ingredients.A study published in the Journal of Food Protection in 2001 cited concerns regarding fungi (the source of mycotoxins) in commercial pet foods and warned about the "risk for animal health".

In 2006, a study published in the Journal of Agricultural and Food Chemistry confirmed mycotoxins in pet foods around the world and concluded that contamination of mycotoxins in pet foods can lead to chronic effects on the health of pets.In 2007, the International Journal of Food Microbiology published a study that claimed "mycotoxin contamination in pet food poses a serious health threat to pets", and listed them: aflatoxins, ochratoxins, trichothecenes, zearalenone, fumonisins and fusaric acid.

A 2008 study published in the Journal of Animal Physiology and Animal Nutrition found high levels of mycotoxins in the raw ingredients used for pet food in Brazil. A 2010 study in the Journal of Mycotoxin Research tested 26 commercial dog foods and found mycotoxins at concerning sub-lethal levels. It was determined that long-term exposure to low levels of confirmed mycotoxins could pose chronic health risks.

For all the above reasons, a trend away from feed ingredients and toward USDA-certified ingredients fit for human consumption has developed. In 1999, another fungal toxin triggered the recall of dry dog food made by Doane Pet Care at one of its plants, including Ol' Roy, Wal-Mart's brand, as well as 53 other brands. This time the toxin killed 25 dogs.

A 2005 consumer alert was released for contaminated Diamond Pet Foods for dogs and cats. Over 100 canine deaths and at least one feline fatality have been linked to Diamond Pet Foods contaminated by potentially deadly aflatoxin, according to Cornell University veterinarians.

Common Mistakes When Cooking For Your Dog

When you don't prepare balanced meals that are individualized to your pet's needs, it can come at a cost. Nutrition deficiency (or excess) can lead to diseases, such as malnutrition or obesity, and can ultimately be fatal.

"Each of the ~40 essential nutrients required by dogs has a specific role in the body. When they are provided in inadequate concentrations, the function is not optimal and suffering may result," explains Dr. Larsen. "Similarly, nutrient excesses can also cause illness. While the impact of an unbalanced diet may be mild and not even noticed or attributed to the diet by the owner, these problems can also be very severe, and pets do not always survive."

- Relying On Multiple Diets To Create "Balance"

"Our study and my clinical experience has demonstrated that this approach is very unlikely to address problems since so many recipes share the same deficiencies," cautions Dr. Larsen.

- Using Unsafe/Unhealthy Ingredients

There is a wide variety of unhealthy and unsafe foods to avoid when preparing meals for your dog. Potentially toxic ingredients are of special concern, including chocolate, xylitol, avocado, grapes, raisins, onions, garlic, and macadamia nuts.

The above list is not exhaustive and other potential issues can arise if you're not careful about ingredients. So make sure to always be aware of which foods are safe for dogs. Additionally, cites Dr. Bartes, a certain type of heart disease called dilated cardiomyopathy has recently been reported in dogs eating homemade diets that are grain-free, legume-based, and high-fiber.

- Not Following Recipes

"Most general recipes provide vague instructions for ingredients or preparation. This leaves the owner to interpret what type of meat to use, or which supplement product to buy," warns Dr. Larson, of the potential difficulty in following dog food recipes.

Rather than improvising, it's important to run any questions by a veterinary nutritionist. That way, you'll be able to understand the impact alternative ingredients might have on your dog.

- Understating the Impact of Dietary Changes

Ideally, when you go about creating a custom recipe for your dog, it will be under the guidance of a board-certified veterinary nutritionist. Factors like your dog's eating history, weight, and overall health should be considered. To make sure the food you're introducing is having the desired impact, you'll want to monitor your pet's health for changes over time.

An Alternative To Home Cooking

"Cooking for your pet is a process that's demanding on your time, labor, space, and finances," says Dr. Larsen. Home cooking is not for everyone, though, and it doesn't have to be. Another option to provide your dog with whole ingredients is to get carefully prepared ready-made meals.

"There are commercial foods that can be purchased that contain whole ingredients that are pre-cooked. Which is very close to cooking," notes Dr. Bartges. So, while you might think that cooking for your dog is better for their health, it can be just as beneficial to purchase pre-prepared food that's made with the same principles in mind. Whichever method you choose, just to make sure you are always catering to your dog's individual health and nutrition needs.

Conclusion

Dogs have managed to adapt over thousands of years to survive on the meat and non-meat scraps and leftovers of human existence and thrive on a variety of foods, with studies suggesting dogs' ability to digest carbohydrates easily may be a key difference between dogs and wolves.

With the increasing number of pet food recalls, many dog lovers are switching from store-bought food to home-cooked meals for their canines. If you're new to this, it might seem overwhelming. You know what to cook for yourself and your family but might be unsure about what to cook for your dog.

Printed in the USA
CPSIA information can be obtained
at www.ICGtesting.com
LVHW052232071224
798586LV00030B/691